Soul Talks

POWER OF INTENTION

ACHARYA SHREE YOGEESH

Siddha Sangh Publications

SIDDHA SANGH PUBLICATIONS
9985 E. Hwy 56, Windom, Texas 75492
info@siddhayatan.org

Copyright © 2020 by Acharya Shree Yogeesh
Compilation/Editing: Sadhvi Siddhali Shree
Cover Design: Sadhvi Anubhuti

www.siddhayatan.org
www.acharyashreeyogeesh.com

ISBN - 1-7334750-1-3
ISBN - 9-781-7334750-1-3

Library of Congress Control Number - 2020946568
Printed in the United States of America.

Disclaimer: Please note that not all exercises, diet plans, or other suggestions,
mentioned in this book are suitable for everyone. This book is not intended to
replace the need for consultation with medical doctors and other professionals.
Before changing any diet, exercise routine, or any other plans discussed in this
book, seek appropriate professional medical advice to ensure it is acceptable for
you. The author and publisher are not responsible for any problems arising from the
use or misuse of the information, materials, demonstrations or references provided
in this book. Results are not guaranteed.

CONTENTS

1 | Your Mind and Intentions

Your soul is infinite, eternal, and powerful. That is who you really are. If you ask others who they are, they will often identify with their mind or thoughts. In the real sense, you cannot identify yourself with that which is unstable and fluctuates back and forth between the past and future. That is not who you are. Because of the mind, because of karma, the soul is weak and stuck. That's why, in this book *Soul Talks: Power of Intention*, I will share with you how to purify your mind so that it helps you on your spiritual journey. You will learn how to make your mind and intentions pure so that you can reach the highest states of consciousness. Without a pure mind, you cannot be free. Once you have a pure mind, then you have the best instrument to help your soul liberate itself.

The mind plays a very strong role in your life. Even though it doesn't physically exist, it has a lot of power to help you or hurt you. It can help you on the spiritual path a lot, it can help you in business, it can help you in understanding your relationships, it can help you excel in education, it can be creative, it might have ideas on how to help others, and in general it can help you be an overall good person. The mind can also destroy you. It has a lot of power — it has ego, anger, greediness, violence, deceitfulness, and can take you down the wrong path. When you are in mind, you resist things, which leads to inner tension, stress and negativity. This is why you may feel you have a lot of problems. You're too much into your mind. If there's no mind, there are no problems. It is better to use your mind as an instrument to help you grow spiritually and liberate yourself versus having your undisciplined mind take you down the wrong path. For the most part, we suffer because of our mind. The whole world can go crazy just because of it.

As soon as the mind senses you are trying to grow spiritually, it will begin to attack you more. It doesn't want to lose its power. It doesn't want your soul to have control. It is the nature of the mind to keep you always on the wrong path creating misery and more problems even though you deeply wish to be on the right one. When you are living in your soul, which is your true self, you may encounter challenges, but you will flow with them. That is why it's important to understand and master your intentions.

Bhāvana means "intention" in Sanskrit, and it lives extremely close to the soul. Your soul is made up of very subtle special particles and the bhāvana is the first layer of substance that surrounds it. It is like the first layer of mind that is closest to the soul. That first layer needs to be pure; however, in reality it probably isn't at this time for you. Your bhāvana plays a very important role in your journey. An intention can make you very happy if it's pure or if it's bad it can make your life miserable. The purest intentions help you progress spiritually and help you to become a great person in the society. How are you the greatest? Because you are the purest one. Where there is purity, you are truly a shining soul! On the other hand, the worst intentions can drag you down and make you burn in hellish planets where there is only suffering. Hellish suffering is not like how we suffer on this earth today. Every single moment, not just minute, the pain level is immense. There is not such a moment where there is peace, relaxation, and relief. It's constant pain. The only time there is a brief moment of relief is when a Tirthankara is born somewhere in the universe.

A Tirthankara is an extraordinary soul who is born with the best particles of the universe as a result of their karma. Typically, a Tirthankara is born at a time where there is a lot of suffering in that society and they bring the necessary teachings to help wake that society up and inspire them to be spiritual. A Tirthankara is not born enlightened; however, that body is their last body and they will be enlightened then liberated. There is no difference between an enlightened master and a Tirthankara except for the extraordinary body they are born with.

The last Tirthankara who was born on this planet lived over 2600 years ago. His name was Tirthankara Mahavira. According to the Samanic Tradition, the oldest spiritual system, Mahavira was the last one out of the 24 Tirthankaras who lived on this planet in this current era.

The Tirthankaras suffer a lot in the beginning of their life.

Even though they are extraordinary, they are not exempt from pain. They are born with three perfect knowledges, *jnanas*: *Matijnana* which is higher intelligence from their senses like visual learning. Their memory is kind of photographic. They don't need to read books. All they have to do is flip through the pages and the knowledge is there. *Shrutijnana* is general knowledge or spiritual knowledge accumulated from their previous lives. And, lastly, *avadhijnana*; they have the ability to see a limited distance with crystal clarity. A very far distance, but still limited. Nothing blocks their vision. They can see through mountains. It's not a physical vision, but instead an inner vision that allows them to see very clearly. Everyone has these abilities too, but they don't know that the power is hidden inside of them and how to access them because their intentions are not pure.

When the Tirthankara leaves the world by renouncing royalty, their luxuries, their relationships, everything, the way they renounce it is quite unique. They are born with so much wealth, and because of their compassion, they donate from morning to evening. They don't stop giving. Whoever comes to them, they give. Not just for one or two days, nor one or two months, but a whole year. This is called *varshi dan.* It means donating for one year continuously. Can you imagine how much money, how much wealth they have? All the poor people become so rich. After a Tirthankara renounces and takes diksha, their mind becomes transparent. There is no reflection. Once this happens, they achieve *manah paryaya jnana* knowledge — they have the ability to read all these particles of everybody's mind. When their mind is pure, or they have no mind, they can see everything clearly. By their own efforts, willpower, and discipline to burn all of their karma, they eventually reach the highest states of consciousness and become enlightened. This is called *keval jnana*. It's at this state they realize fully that there are twelve intentions that have to be purified.

In this *Soul Talks*, you will learn about the 12 bhāvanas or intentions, so you can begin improving them little by little. You don't want to go to a hellish planet. It is so unbearably painful. It is better to use this life to progress and not to digress. That's why you need to always do your best to keep your intention, mind, speech, and actions pure. When the intention is impure, the mind is impure, everything is dirty and muddy. Like if someone wears glasses, if there is mud on their glasses, they cannot see through. But if their glasses are very clean, they can see clearly.

The power of intention can destroy your *bhava*, which means your "cycle of birth and death." People continue to suffer because they are born and then they die. Death is painful and people become unconscious as a result of the pain experienced. There is pain in birth too. And, the human life, and really all forms of life, always has some kind of suffering. No matter what. No one has a perfect life. If you are a human being, you will suffer. Never think others do not suffer even though they may appear to have a perfect life. Maybe they are not physically suffering, but how do you know that they are not suffering emotionally and mentally? Even angels are not free from suffering. They know they must come back to be a human in order to liberate themselves. That's why it is incredibly important to work on yourself, to work on your intention, and to free yourself from the cycle of birth and death.

Awareness is the key to understanding the mind. This is not easy. Why? Because the mind doesn't exist. If it exists, you can understand it. It doesn't have a structure to touch and feel it. We don't know if the mind is heavy or light in weight. We don't know if the mind is hot or cold, smooth or rough. We don't know because we are unable to touch it, see it, smell it, taste it, or hear it. It's amazing, isn't it? Something we cannot physically experience rules over our lives and creates chaos.

According to Western thought, there are three types of mind: conscious, subconscious, and unconscious. I would add higher conscious to this as well. The conscious mind is more of general awareness, while the subconscious is a state of sometimes being aware and not aware. Most people live in a subconscious state. This mind is always confused. The unconscious mind is deep and sleeping. Sometimes when the unconscious begins to wake up, you can get connected with direct knowing. Higher consciousness is attained through waking up the unconscious mind. All these types of consciousness are still considered dravya manas, lower mind.

To help us understand the mind, the Samanic Tradition divides it into two parts. First is *dravya manas* and the second is *bhāva manas*. Dravya manas is like a gross mind. People get angry, violent, or blow up because of the gross mind. They can go so far with their anger and kill others. They have no control because they never tried to understand what the mind is. Dravya manas is a very kind of heavy mind which is closer to your physical body. You can even say it is like the shadow of your physical body. The shadow is the closest thing to you, but if you try and catch it, you won't be able to. When you run after it, the shadow runs faster than you. When you run the fastest you can run, it is still ahead of you. The dravya manas mind, which serves as an ideology, has a structure and does exist. The lower mind holds all your beliefs, faith, culture, religion, ideas, etc. The lower mind can be caught and measured with advanced technology, but the higher mind, bhāva manas, cannot be examined with science.

In truth, the mind doesn't exist. It seems confusing, doesn't it? The real mind, bhāva manas mind, does not exist. Physically, that is.

Bhāva manas means "instrument to know the subtlest reality" and it is the layer of mind closest to the soul. This type of mind does not have a reflection; therefore, it's uncatchable. I call bhāva manas "higher mind" or "pure mind." Bhāva manas is still mind. And the mind is still garbage compared to the soul. Even still, the bhāva manas will not take you astray if you live by it. The dravya manas mind, on the other hand, cannot be trusted. That is why you have difficulty trusting yourself and you are full of fear and negative thoughts. The dravya manas mind is ruling you and not the bhāva manas. If you know how to use the bhāva manas, you can get connected to right and higher knowing. All fears, negativities, and such non-sense will leave you.

The 12 bhāvanas, intentions, which I will share with you in this book, reside in the bhāva manas. The bhāva manas is very difficult to understand or experience because of its subtleness. You need to lift yourself so high that you are in a higher state of consciousness to understand bhāva manas. Dravya manas is much easier to grasp and absorb since it's more gross. Psychology and medicine try to study, work with, and understand the gross mind. But no science can measure bhāva manas.

Here's an example of how to understand the mind. On the surface of the ocean, the waves are choppy, there is a lot of noise, the waves are high and low. This is the dravya manas mind. If you go deeper into the ocean, it is very quiet and it doesn't move at all. This is bhāva manas. In meditation, most people find a little peace just a little bit below the surface of mind. But when they get in touch with the bhāva manas, it is totally different. There are no thoughts and activities in the mind. It's a beautiful space. Then with more understanding, practice, concentration, and the ability to relax, you can go deeper and deeper and touch the very bottom of the ocean — soul.

Another example. Imagine there is a water stream with a hundred people crossing it. All the sand particles spread across the water which makes the stream look dirty. But after all the people are out of the water, the sand begins to settle and the water becomes crystal clear. Dravya manas is all those floating particles, which makes the mind active and dirty. When the sand settles and there is clarity and calmness, that is bhāva manas.

Until enlightenment happens, an advanced soul will always be in bhāva manas. The closer to enlightenment someone is, they can see what the soul is like, but not really 100% know it. You can never get a taste of the direct soul until you are enlightened. Up until that point you are tasting the flavor of the soul through your bhāva manas.

It's easy to talk about spirituality when you have touched bhāva manas or are in it because you are in mind. But when you are in soul, you cannot talk, you don't want to talk. A master has the ability to consciously switch between which state they are in - in soul, in bhāva manas, or dravya manas. Disciples and students are the ones who push the master to talk when they are in the soul state. Then the master will use their bhāva manas or dravya manas to communicate.

Gautam Swami, Tirthankara Mahavira's chief disciple, was the one pushing him to talk. Because of his effort a lot of the teachings were saved and continue to help people today. I personally do not write these books by hand. My disciples are the ones transcribing what I say; they push me to speak! When I give lectures, satsangs, and discourses, I'm using bhāva manas. When I am discussing let's say construction or math, I'm using dravya manas. When I am silent, I'm with soul. You will experience the difference.

The real power inside of you is your soul. This is what you need to get connected with. Learn how to bypass your mind and be in soul.

One student went to the philosopher/mystic Gurdjieff. Although he was strange, people of that time considered him to be a spiritual master in the western countries. The student asked Gurdjieff if he could guide him. He said he was a seeker, a searcher. Gurdjieff invited the student to an evening event. As soon as the student arrived, Gurdjieff offered him a bottle of alcohol.

"I don't drink," the student declined.

"Do you want to learn?"

"Yes, of course."

"Then drink."

They both were drunk and their whole body was loose. Physically, everything was loose — the muscles, tissues, nervous system, everything. This is a fragile state of mind. It's almost bhāva manas. If you say something to someone and they are in this kind of state, it could fully trigger that person. Whatever that person is holding, it will be released through shouting, screaming, or even violence.

Four hours passed and they were both extremely drunk. Someone took the student home and dropped him off to get rest. The next morning, Gurdjieff called the student who didn't remember anything from the night before.

"How are you?"

"Ok. Can I come back to learn?"

"Of course, I can teach you. Now I know who you are. Before I didn't know who you are and I learned you have a lot of anger and violence inside of you. I cannot teach you if I don't know you. Now I understand what to teach you."

You cannot really teach or help a person if you don't know what they are holding inside. If they are holding a lot of emotions, all those emotions will rise to the surface. I don't support Gurdjieff's methods. He was a strange teacher, but that was his way.

14

Gurdjieff used to invite students over to his house for parties. He would serve them wine and when he would toast he'd say, "Cheers to the idiots!" People wondered which idiots he was toasting to. The mind is the idiot. The mind can be your best friend or worst enemy. You have to understand that the mind is like a language. The mind is an ideology. And the mind gets the "words" from your senses.

Your ears will hear something. Your eyes will see something. The information received through your senses will pass on to your nervous system where your nerves will then carry that message to your brain where it is processed. The brain is a structure. It is an organ. It has no intelligence. Your senses don't have intelligence either. Your eyes see, but they don't interpret what they see. Your ears hear, but your ears do not interpret what you've heard. The senses are like a servant. Your physical body, your senses, your nervous system, and your brain are all like employees. The question is, employees of whom? Your brain has no intelligence, so that is not the answer. Therefore, they are employees of your mind, bhāva manas, which contains your intelligence. It is almost like a reflection of you as your body has a shadow.

It has little intelligence, but doesn't really know anything. That bhāva manas passes the message to your soul. Because your soul is weak, it accepts whatever messages are received from the senses and mind as truth. However, the truth is, once you purify your senses and once you purify your mind, your soul will not be enslaved to the senses and mind. Instead they will work for the soul. But because the soul has been wandering in suffering, is weak, and full of pain, it cannot see clearly. The mind itself does not have intelligence, only the power behind it has the intelligence, and that is the soul.

If you think about it, when a person dies, their senses are dead, their organs are dead, and their mind is gone, what remains is their soul. The soul, because of karma, will be born again with a new set of senses, a new body, and a new mind.

What Gurdjieff was trying to teach was that your sense and mind were the idiots — they have no intelligence. The real power is with Soul.

Recently, a student asked a question during her Meditation Retreat with me. She said, "I don't know what happened to me. I've never meditated before and when I closed my eyes I felt like there was a flood of light. Is it real?"

I asked, "Did you try to meditate?"

"No."

"When meditation happens naturally like that, it is real. When you force meditation then your mind can make up things."

"What was the light?"

"Your soul is trying to wake up and it won't until you begin to understand. You need to purify your mind to understand."

Purification of the mind is necessary to move towards living in higher states of consciousness and understanding the power of intention. You need to learn how to purify your gross mind, dravya manas to bhāva manas. People mostly live in dravya manas. The mind is readable. It's full of thoughts. There is nothing special about this gross mind. However, when you have purified your mind and begin to live in bhāva manas, then that is the best thing for you. Bhāva manas is not a readable mind. Bhāva manas is blank. Enlightenment is blank. When a person is enlightened, they are in a way in a state of nothingness and everythingness. In order for enlightened masters to connect with others on the human/mind level, they need to actually disconnect from their soul (state of blankness/ nothingness) and use the gross mind in order to read other people's mind, or learn a language, or even to speak and connect with other people. That's why sometimes it's difficult for enlightened ones to teach or to share, because if they are constantly in the soul state, they are unable to speak because they are in the infinite. If their dravya manas mind is uneducated or illiterate, then that master will be unable to teach — at least with words.

The few masters that exist today mostly don't speak. It doesn't mean that he or she is not enlightened. Enlightenment has nothing to do with the mind, their level of intelligence or knowledge, because those things belong to the lower mind. However, if a person is educated or knows languages prior to their enlightenment, then they can use that mind as a tool. An enlightened person is not necessarily perfect nor should they be judged to be. They have a body (a machine), a brain structure, and sometimes the human body makes mistakes (like a computer), but it doesn't take away from their own realization of the soul.

Here's an example of what enlightened masters can go through. Pretend you are on stage and you see one hundred people in the room. Unless you focus on a single person, you will always see 100 people in the room. In some way, an enlightened master is connected to the whole universe and they see the universe as a whole; however, if they need to find a little child in America, they will need to refocus from looking at the universe, find the planet Earth, zoom into the United States, zoom in more to go to the specific state the child is in, and eventually find the little child. It is a process to go from universe to specific. Like Google maps. Usually, you start at the bird's eye view, then you zoom in to find the location you are looking for. It is a process. Enlightened masters have to go to a lower level of mind to be with people and to live in the world. In an instant, they are connected and see the universe. It's quite fascinating. Enlightenment is unexplainable in many ways.

Experiencing self-realization, attaining enlightenment, connecting with soul are all possible for you. To say it will happen in this lifetime for you depends on your karma and efforts. It's not guaranteed. To move towards this spiritual goal, you need to purify the mind and you need to stop being a slave to your senses and your mind. This is not easy. Your bhāva manas is a slave to your dravya manas. How does that happen? Let me explain.

Let's say there is a King and he has many employees and because the King has bad habits he often gets drunk and ends up sleeping all day. How can a King run a successful Kingdom and be strong and powerful if he's drunk or asleep all day? It's when the King becomes weak the employees begin to take over. No one is giving them direction. They do their job, then their mind gets corrupt, then instead of being humble employees they become egoistic. Eventually, they become strong and powerful and they begin to rule the Kingdom, not the King. Your mind, brain, nervous system, and senses are your employees and they have taken over your soul. You allowed them to take over because you lacked discipline. You enjoy your pleasures, you enjoy your lust, you enjoy love, you are too much into attachment, you have so many desires, you get affected by little things, your ego is big or your self-esteem is too low…all of these and many more things have made you a slave. You are a soul. You are powerful. You are intelligent. You are timeless. Yet you are not. Because of your weaknesses you do not live in soul. You do not live in the present moment. You go up and down. You are imbalanced. You are like the roaring waves of the ocean, not calm, not peaceful, not still. The main question is, how to be in charge again? How to be in control? How to have your employees work with you and not overtake you?

The mind is dirty. The mind is corrupt. The mind is full of pollution. That's why it's not easy to purify the mind. But what you need to do is start flooding your mind with positive thoughts. Your mind loves and thrives on negativity. It loves fear. It loves chaos. It likes imbalance. It enjoys misery. When you begin to have a strong mind, in a positive way, then it works for you and not against you. In 24 hours, a person has around 60,000 thoughts. Most people's thoughts are very negative. Negative minds create a negative world and that's why this world and all living beings in it suffer. Negative minds create chaos, negative minds create disease, negative minds are a major

21

disturbance. Sometimes people get so negative it doesn't leave them for years. Nobody can help a negative person because their negativity is so powerful. Unfortunately, negative people drag down other people, and I don't doubt that you've experienced that kind of person in your life. Or, maybe you were the one who brought someone else down?

All emotions are negative forces. Pure and positive emotions like compassion and love can still drag you down and make you lost. That's why it's better to get out of all emotions, get out of your mind, and live in soul. How do emotions make you lost? Here's an example:

A long time ago, Catholic monks and nuns used to carry ropes when they would walk village to village. When they came across a well or pond and an animal or human fell down, they would assist and rescue them, take them out, with the hope they are still alive. The people used to think these monks and nuns were compassionate. They knew that these wells were deep and animals or humans would be unable to climb out, so it was very kind of the monks and nuns to try and help them. Every time they visited a well they would check to see if something was inside. If it was empty, then they couldn't save the animal or human. They used to think, "How can we go to heaven if we are not saving creatures?" It shows deep down that maybe they wanted an animal or human trapped so that they can perform the rescue and receive the virtues. They secretly wanted them to fall so that they can be able to save. Even a pure emotion like love and compassion can be corrupt. Very rarely can you find pure love.

There was once a married couple who had a child that was six years old. For the most part, their marriage was loving, but something eventually happened between them. One day, the man came back from work and told his wife he wanted a divorced.

"Are you serious?" she asked.

"I know we've been together for 20 years, but yes, I want a divorce."

"Ok, I will divorce you, but you need to do one thing and then I will gladly sign the papers."

"Ok, what is it?"

"I want you to carry me from the bedroom to the kitchen for the next 30 days, as you used to carry me when we first got married. I don't have any other desire."

"I will give you money instead," he replied because he was in love with another lady.

"I don't need your money. Just do this one thing."

He agreed. He also arranged with his girlfriend that he would be unable to see her for one month because he made an agreement with his wife with the promise that she'll sign the divorce papers.

The man would go to work, they would sleep together, and when he woke up he would carry his wife through the door and bring her back to the kitchen before he goes to work. Their child became so happy seeing this. Every day, he would pick her up and the child was always excited to see them that way. The child even inspired his dad to say "I love you" as he would bring the wife down to the bed. After a week, the husband began to hug and kiss her before leaving. The child became even happier. This became the routine for two weeks and suddenly the man began to have feelings for his wife again. He also noticed her body was becoming lighter and weaker but didn't say anything.

After the third week, his feelings grew stronger and he began to see the woman he used to love deeply. He remembered how much she would take care of him and the family. All of the feelings flooded him. He remembered how his child would always cry seeing them argue, but now his son was so happy. Eventually, it was the last night of his promise. He went to his girlfriend to tell her that he fell back in love with his wife again and that he will not seek a divorce. When he returned home, he found an emotional letter:

"I wanted you to pick me up every day because I knew our son would be happy to see us together. I also didn't want him to know that I had cancer."

The doctor gave her a month to live and she died.

The point of the story is this: Worldly love, which is often corrupted love (and the most common), can become pure love if you learn how to practice it.

Compassion can be corrupted. Love can be corrupted. If it can be corrupted, then it was never pure. Pure love has no boundaries. It's like sunshine and it shines everywhere. There are no conditions. If you want to purify your mind, you first need to see what is hidden beneath it and what is disturbing or bothering your mind and causing it to become corrupt. Is it power? Or emotions? You have to be clear with those things. Analyze yourself to see the pollution and corruption in your mind. Clearing the mind is not an easy thing to do. What you can remind yourself is that if you do not work on your mind and its impurities, you will be dragged through suffering. You cannot go through the process of experiencing the 12 bhāvanas, levels of intention, unless you understand and work on your mind. Going through the 12 bhāvanas reflects your journey of purifying the mind and you will learn all about this next.

2 | The 12 Levels of Intention

The bhāva manas mind is like a reflection of the soul. Even though the soul is bodiless, shapeless, formless, the bhāva manas acts like a shadow to the soul. Pure intention lives in the bhāva manas mind. Pure intention is when your mind is lighter and when your mind is not burdened, corrupt, or polluted. A good example of bhāva manas is to see the mind like a mirror or prism which uses a crystal kind of glass. Whatever you place in front of a prism, like a flower, you will see the flower inside the prism even though the flower is not inside the actual glass. Bhāva manas is like that. The soul is near the bhāva manas, it's not inside it, but the bhāva manas prism reflects the soul in the purest way. You cannot see it, experience it, or understand the bhāva manas or the soul if your dravya manas is impure. Most people live in the dravya manas. That's why they experience so many difficulties in life. Their mind is polluted. A person can be very intelligent, but if their mind is impure, they can misuse their intelligence due to the pollution and bad intentions of the dravya manas mind.

Intention refers to the way you think. People can think in negative or bad ways or people can think in good ways too. Sometimes your intention is not to hurt someone, but the person gets hurt anyways. If this is the case, you don't collect much karma because your intention is pure. However, if you are unaware or your intention is impure and you hurt someone by yelling, screaming, or name-calling, then you will collect karma.

Karma are particles that cover and block the soul and its light, which makes you live in illusion, wander in the world, go through pain, suffering, joy, and it keeps you in the cycle of birth and death. Your real goal is supposed to be karma-free. Soul, by itself, is karma free; however, it is surrounded by dark clouds of ignorance just as clouds can block the sun's shine. The clouds don't touch the sun, but they are dense and dark enough to block its light.

When you have negative or violent thoughts, actions and speech towards any living being, you will collect bad karma. If you are trying to save a bug, like a creature falling into a lake, and you try to rescue it and it happens to still die, you will not collect karma because your intention was not to kill, but to save. You can also collect good karma too, like when you help people but deep down inside you are seeking some kind of reward, praise, or recognition. It means you didn't help wholeheartedly and selflessly so it brings you good karma.

Yes, it can help you enjoy life a little bit better, but good karma keeps you in the cycle of birth and death too. It is best to be bad and good karma free. That's what liberation means. When you have impure intentions, it will bring you bad karma. But pure intention can burn your karma, and that is why I'm sharing this 12-level system of intention with you so you know what you need to purify and how, so that you can one day be free.

A saint was bathing in the river and he saw a scorpion drowning in the water. The saint felt so much compassion for the scorpion and thought to himself, "I'd better save him, otherwise he will drown!" With no protective gloves, he scooped up the scorpion out of the water with his bare hands. The scorpion stung him right away. The saint fell down because of the strong and painful bite. He thought again, "He's still drowning and he's going to die! I better save him." He picked him up again and the scorpion stung him again. The scorpion fell back in the water.

A young man who was witnessing the saint approached him at the river. "Can I ask you a question?"

"Yes, of course," he replied.

"If this scorpion is stinging you, why do you want to save him?"

The saint answered, "Look, my nature is to save and this little creature's nature is to sting. My body is 6 ft tall. Look at his tiny little body. If this little creature does not want to leave its nature, which is to bite, then why should I leave my nature which is to save? I want to save it."

The saint tried again and was successful and put the scorpion back on land.

This is called pure intention. As you begin to live a purer life, your intention becomes purer and purer, and then your pure mind becomes the best instrument for your soul. It will change your life.

The human mind is not the only mind that is impure. Animals and other creatures have a mind too. There is a type of little fish, the size of rice, called Tandul Matsya that lives on a whale's head. It's like lice for whales. When a whale is hungry, it opens its big mouth and swallows a bunch of fish, not all but most. It doesn't really catch fish because the fish just swim inside. Meanwhile, this little head louse creature, which has five senses and a mind, watches the whale and thinks to itself, "This whale has no sense. A thousand fish come into his mouth and he lets them go. If I had this big body I would not let even one escape." Now this little louse cannot eat fish, but day and night he curses the whale, collecting bad karma for being consumed with impure intentions and negative thoughts. He cannot eat fish, but he wants to eat them. He cannot kill, but he wants to kill. This louse can collect so much bad karma within a very small period of time because it doesn't have a long life span. It maybe has a lifetime of a hundred days or so. 24 hours a day in these kinds of bad thoughts and intentions makes the louse collect so much bad karma to the degree it can send it to a hellish planet.

We need to have a purified mind. Purification of the mind is very important because the mind is corrupt and brings a lot of sin and karma. Karma is not easy to break. Do your best to keep your intention pure even when negative thoughts attack you.

One king asked Tirthankara Mahavira, "Kaham chare. Kaham chitthe. Kaham ase. Kaham saye. Kaham bujanto bhasanto, pavv kammam na bhandai."

Master, can you tell me how to walk? How to sit? How to sleep? How to eat? How to talk? How to do everything without collecting any sin or bad karma? Can you give me the technique please?

He said, "Very easy. Jayam chare. Jayam chitthe. Jayam ase. Jayam saye. Jayam bujanto bhasanto, pavv kammam na bhandai."

Walk with awareness. Sit with awareness. Sleep with awareness. Eat with awareness. Talk with awareness. When you do everything with awareness you will not collect bad karma.

When you walk, walk with pure intention. Walk with awareness. What if there's a creature crawling and you step on it? You will kill it. If you are on awareness duty, at least you are looking forward and seeing three steps ahead of you so that there are more chances you will not crush any living being. Being on duty means you have awareness to watch your step and not to kill anything. Sometimes, even by walking with awareness and you try to save the creature or not crush it, by accident it still gets killed. Your intention while on duty was to save, so you won't collect any karma. If you are on duty with a pure intention, you cannot collect karma. If you are not on duty, even if nothing happens, you are still collecting karma because you are not aware and your intention is not there. If your thoughts are to protect life, you are on duty. If someone isn't on duty, they don't care and they are fully unaware.

The degree of karma collected depends on your intention. Intention is the main thing which can destroy all of your karma, burn all of your karma, and ultimately end your death and birth cycle. Intention is important and is like a fire. If you have mountain-high-like karma on your soul, just one little pure intention can burn that whole mountain quickly. It might take a few days, but it can bring that whole mountain of karma down. We do have trillions and trillions of layers of karma mountains covering the soul, so it takes time to burn everything down. As soon as you begin to live with awareness and pure intention, those layers will burn quickly and no more karmic layers will be added.

The 12-level system of intention serves as a guide and instrument to help you to understand what pure intention really is. They are like reflections and contemplations that show you where you stand. Are your intentions pure, impure, or are they mixed? Are you mostly pure or mostly impure or equally both? When you know where you are at then you know what areas you need to improve on. This is how you grow spiritually and purify yourself more and more.

When you think about your own life while learning about these intentions, you need to be honest with yourself. Think about the degree of how pure or impure your intentions are. It's easy to show off to others how pure you are. You can lie to others, but you cannot lie to yourself because you know the truth. I see this often with new-age people or people who consider themselves "yogis" and "spiritual teachers." Human beings can be very good actors. They can pretend to others and the blind people will accept them, but in the real sense one cannot run away from the truth and reality. The karma will be there, the illusion will cloud them, and they will suffer because of their illusion. A master can see right through them. It's a thick cloud around their soul. Work on yourself because you want to be better. Don't do spiritual work to impress others or feel better about yourself when people praise you. Focus on yourself. Don't focus on other people. Instead of increasing your ego, work on liberating your soul.

The following are the 12 levels of intention:

1. *Anitya Bhāvana*. *Anitya* means "impermanence of the world." If you live with the intention, mindset, and awareness that there is nothing permanent about this world or your life, you will begin to live in a higher state of thinking. Whether challenges, pain, or suffering arises you know it will pass and will be less affected by it compared to others. No one is permanent. Birth guarantees death. If things are permanent, then everything stays forever. That's why if things are temporary, why not do good with your life? If we know that we will die one day, why hang on to grudges, negativity, or take revenge? Why have heart attacks over loss of money, people, or other things? There is no need to be jealous, be hateful, or be mean if there is impermanence. There's a level of freedom when you live with the mindset that everything is impermanent because you will not be taken or affected by things and you will practice non-attachment.

When you live with the anitya bhāvana intention, you are automatically away from violence, negativity, hatred, ego, or anger. Why have ego or anger? For what? You will not last forever. Why are you holding on to these things? Why are you allowing these things to control you? They are impermanent too!

In a way, we are lucky we are not permanent here. Every time we are born we get a new start. Most people don't remember their past lives and sometimes that is a good thing. It gives everyone a fresh start. A new body. A new mind. A new chance. It's a new beginning. Learning to live in a spiritual way is like a fresh start. Learning to let go and be free. When we live with the intention of impermanence, we are free.

Time passes quickly, so that's why I suggest you use the rest of your life wisely. Forget if you wasted it or not up until this point, the next moment is new. That's the best thing. Every day is a special day. Every moment is a new and special moment. So much awaits you to experience. A bliss that's indescribable, but you need to wake up. Use the rest of your life to wake up. Live with pure thoughts and intention. When you do so, you won't be attached or taken by the world. You'll be less into the desires. You will help others more and that is one of the best ways to burn all of your karma.

2. *Asharan Bhāvana*. *Asharan* means "no one can protect or save you." It is our illusion that others can protect or save someone from death. Everyone must die and no one can protect or save you from the fate. Even if a child is dying, a father or mother can't save her. When it's a soul's time, it is their time. No one can interfere with that. Someone can build the strongest castle to protect them from death, but no matter what death will find you. It doesn't care how much money you have, how much knowledge you have, how famous you are, or how loved and respected you are by the family and community, when the time is up, it is time to go.

When you live with this kind of intention, you will realize that the only thing that can save your soul is spirituality. Spirituality is your protection. Spirituality is like an island in the middle of nowhere and after crossing the ocean of suffering it becomes your shelter and safety.

Living with this intention also teaches you to be independent, to be responsible for your life, to be strong and confident. The stronger you are within, because you cannot rely on anyone to protect or save you, you become so strong for the path. That strength is what helps you to stay focused, driven, inspired, and to stay on the spiritual track towards enlightenment and freedom.

3. *Samsaar Bhāvana. Sansaar* means "the world," in general. The world that you see. You can look at the world the way you want to look at it or you can look at it the right way. When you have pure intention, you have right vision. When you have right vision, you see things as they truly are in the absolute sense. Samsaar bhāvana

is the intention of when you reflect on the world and the suffering that comes along with it. When you reflect about the suffering of yourself and others, it can inspire you to be on the spiritual path so that you begin to transform your life so that you come out of the suffering. One day, you become liberated so you don't have to suffer anymore.

There are so many types of suffering. There's physical suffering, emotional suffering, mental suffering, and spiritual suffering. Each type has many dimensions and many degrees of pain. For someone suffering spiritually, maybe they are so desperate and thirsty to find and discover the Truth, but they are not at peace because they are unable to find the way to the path. There is no one in the world that likes and enjoys suffering. And a lot of the suffering comes from our relationships with others — especially family because we are attached to them. We have to remember relationships are also not permanent. When we die and are born again, we will have a new family.

Can you imagine how many times you have been born and died and how many families you've been a part of?

How can you suffer from the loss of your father or mother, brother or sister in this life, yet you have survived such losses millions of times? It's not to say you're not supposed to grieve, but when you have an understanding of how many relationships you have had in this life and in your past lives, it doesn't make sense to get stuck on one relationship and suffer so greatly. Understanding is key to releasing yourself from illusion.

Here's one Truth you may not know: Every living being has at least seven relationships or connections with every other living being in this universe. So the stranger on the street that you saw while driving, may have been your best friend hundreds of lives ago. Maybe you'll feel something inside when you see that stranger as if you knew them, but you'll continue your life. Every single living being has met the rest of the other living beings in the universe at least seven times. "Soul mates" are souls you tend to stick around more and have closer connections to. They're like deep consistent connections across your lives. Sometimes we remember, but most of the time we forget our connections across the millions and millions of years. Close relationships, we remember better. So who is to say who your real mother is, your real father, your real brother or real sister? You've had many. In the end, we need to remember that this world is full of suffering and pain, there is no need to stay here longer, for what?

When you live with Sansaar intention, your attachment to the world and people will become less. Who to hate, who to be jealous of, who to get angry with and why? No one belongs to you and you don't belong to anyone. When you live with that intention you stop holding onto the world. We think the world is holding us and bringing us the suffering, but really it's because we are holding onto the world and others as to why we suffer.

4. *Ekaatva Bhāvana.* *Ekaatva* refers to "you, yourself," as a soul alone. You are born by yourself and you will die by yourself. No one is born with you and no one will die with you. Everything is you and you alone. Ekaatva bhāvana is having the intention of solitude of soul. You might have family, friends, co-workers, colleagues, associates, but again, in the beginning and end it's you alone. Why get so attached to others that you give them your power and permission to bring you down? Why do you let their criticism and judgement make you upset? It means you don't believe in yourself, even though in the end it's you.

The body you have is not even you. Your mind is not you. Your name is not you. The money you have is not you. What I always share when I teach the Awakening the Soul Retreat is the universal law: That which is given to you is not you. You are a soul. You have always been a soul. Everything else is impermanent, temporary and not the real you. So with this intention, it is better to learn to dissolve your labels, your identities, and to know yourself as a soul more. When you know your soul, you know everything. No one else can give you such realization or knowledge except yourself. Not even a guru or master. In the end, you have to realize everything on your own. Right guidance is important, yes, but in the end it is you. In the end, you must make the final jump to the other side of liberation — bliss. When you live with ekaatva bhāvana, you will stop getting yourself stuck into this world of suffering. It's not easy, but it is a very pure intention.

5. *Anyatva Bhāvana. Anyatva* is "separateness" or "distinctiveness." It's the realization that "I'm not you and

you are not me. We are two individual beings. Our bodies are different, our karma is different." There is no one soul that is exactly like another soul because of karma.

People have the illusion of oneness, they'll claim "Oh, we are one!" No, we are separate. Yes, these people may be in love, but they are still two separate souls. Feeling oneness with all living beings is called non-violence. You feel oneness, but you are not one in the literal sense with all living beings. You are a separate drop in the ocean. You can feel others, but you are not others.

What you sow so shall you reap. If you do good works, you as an individual will get good karma. If you do bad deeds, then you will get the bad result. If your father or mother donates to a church or temple, they will get the good karma result, not the children. Unless it was the children who inspired the parents to donate and give, then the children will also receive a good result because they inspired someone who may not have otherwise given.

Knowing your separateness is important and living in that state of intention. If you are hungry or thirsty, you will need to feed yourself. People pray to God for food, and then food happens to be there, then it is your responsibility to get your own spoon and put the spoon in your mouth. God or anyone else cannot do this for you. It is a misbelief that God does things for you. No. You have to see your own separateness. You need to be responsible. You need to use your body to take care of you. When you understand and see yourself as separate, then you will suffer less.

6. Aʃhuchi Bhāvana. *Aʃhuchi* means "impure" and ashuchi bhāvana is "living with the intention knowing that your body is impure." No matter what you do, your body will be dirty. It doesn't matter how much soap you use or the amount of soap you put into your hair or how much you keep it clean, your body will always be impure. We are lucky that we have skin to cover our bones, tissues, muscles, and blood. If there is no skin, the smell is so bad. When anyone goes to the toilet and relieves themselves, whether it's urine or a bowel movement, what is released smells. Having no skin, you would smell that smell all the time. People release gas, people yawn, burp, sneeze, and the smell can be very bad sometimes. Even family members lose patience and tolerance with someone else's smell or poor hygiene. So no matter how much you try to make your body smell good or perfect, it will always be dirty.

When you wake up sometimes you have something dirty in your eyes, or saliva (drool) came out while you slept, and sometimes you have a runny nose. Having ashuchi bhāvana helps you to not focus so much on your body in the sense that you put makeup, creams, perfumes, and colognes to mask your body because you realize the body itself is impure. People spend a lot of money getting plastic surgery, botox, going to med spas, and doing these kinds of things. It will never stop for them because they are too much into the body. Why waste that money? Yes, it's ok to take care of your body, do your best to keep it clean, and have best hygiene practices so that you don't get sick or make others sick, but really there is no need to be too much into the body. It is dirty. Why don't you work on yourself, instead, to purify yourself so that you live in soul? Your soul doesn't care about makeup or plastic surgery. Learn to be happy with your body. Accept it. Be healthy.

What you can do, which you will learn later in the book,

is to purify your body. It is a good system because you are purifying negativities and toxins stored in your body which creates an impure mind causing you trouble. This is an internal cleanse. When you are clean on the inside, then your external body will glow and shine naturally.

Use your body instead to grow spiritually. It is the best instrument you have. Instead of taking two hours to get ready and put make-up on, take a shower, get ready quickly, and use that extra time to do your spiritual practices. That makes more sense. Because of illusion we prioritize our body in the wrong way. We need to shift our thinking and use our body as a tool to grow spiritually, not to be accepted or to impress other people in society. When you live for soul, you will be happy. When you live for your body, you will be unhappy. Lift yourself higher instead. Remember your body is impure, so it's best to live in soul — the purest thing. Your essence. The real you.

If you don't work on your intentions and don't understand the bhāvanas, you will continue to wander and suffer in this world. The way out of this world of suffering is through the power of intention.

7. Ashrava Bhāvana. Ashrava means "inflow of karmic particles" that goes towards your soul. In every moment, unless you are aware and you have pure intention, karmic particles are always flowing towards you, whether you are positive or negative. The amount of karmic particles flowing towards you depends on your intention. Like I mentioned before, karma is like clouds covering the sun, but in this case it covers from above you, to the left, to the right, and below you. A total of 360. If your sunlight is surrounded by thick clouds, how can it shine? It has so much power, yet seemingly nothing at all. That's why when you live with these intentions or reflections in mind you can burn through the karmic clouds. Why? Because you are on duty and living with higher intention which will not only stop you from collecting karma, you will begin to burn it. Ashrava bhāvana refers specifically to the inflow of karmic particles. When you live with this intention, you are truly practicing awareness because you instantly become aware if there is a negative thought, emotion, or reaction within you. You don't want more karmic particles to flow towards you so your awareness instantly stops it, or switching to positive thoughts instantly stops negative karmic inflow. It takes practice, but practice turns into good awareness habits. Eventually, it will become effortless to always be aware.

Here's a little story: One day, the sun was setting down and it said, "Look, I will be gone one day and nobody can make the light anymore for the earth. Without me there is no light!" Suddenly, one little candle came out semi-confidently, "Hey, I will try my best! I can finish this dark! Don't worry about it if you go, Sun. I will be here and try." This shows the candle thinks very little of itself. It will try, but it is not confident. But a candle does have that kind of power to finish the dark. If you are in a very dark room and a candle is lit, hope is there.

We need to know our power. Enlightenment is difficult to achieve, but it is there, it is within. With enlightenment nothing is really achieved. It's more unveiled or revealed. Your power is not visible yet, but it doesn't mean it's not there. The little candle can destroy the darkness of a big room. We have to be confident in our power. When that power comes, and becomes really strong, then the karma will not flow towards you anymore. When you are strong, and by chance get negative, the positive will take over you and block the karma from coming in. You need to better yourself and make yourself strong. Your soul's nature is not to be weak. It is the most powerful thing.

If you are in a negative mood, angry mood, holding grudges or have jealousy and everything is suppressed and shoved down within you, it will begin to build pressure. That pressure needs to be released somehow. Every volcano erupts because of the pressure. That kind of inner pressure leads to nervous breakdowns, panic and anxiety attacks, and severe mental health issues. We live in a society where it is the norm or expectation to stay silent and never release our emotions. We need to shift these ideas and applaud emotional expression. We need to listen and respect others when they express themselves and release their emotions and make others feel safe, just like we would want to be treated. Releasing emotions is a very vulnerable state, but if we learn how to be better with ourselves and others, our society will become so much better.

People have nervous breakdowns because all emotions are stuffed down into the pit of their stomach. The emotions fester there — anger, fear, guilt, shame and it's not a good feeling. There is no peace, joy, or contentment. Who wants to live that way forever? Learn to be strong to digest bad news. We like to celebrate good news, but we have to be equal to bad news as well. It's easy and pleasant to hear only the good. We only like the good stuff. When you learn to be neutral and unaffected, then you begin to live with peace.

Practicing the Āshrava bhāvana is helpful to create instant awareness as soon as negativities or bad thoughts come to you. Once you are aware you will choose to replace your negative thoughts with positive thoughts because you want to be happy and that it's not worth it to keep on collecting more karma. Ultimately, you are responsible for what affects you and how you react. Learn to replace your anger with happiness. Wake up every day and choose happiness. You really have two choices, to be happy or unhappy. Choose happiness.

8. Samvar Bhāvana. *Samvar bhāvana* refers to "how to stop the inflow of karma." Ashrava bhāvana refers to being aware that there is an inflow of karma; however, samvar bhāvana is knowing how to stop the karma from coming in. Samvar bhāvana means to stop the bad thoughts, negativities, jealousy, hate, ego, violence, etc. from entering you. It is very important to stop all these negativities, otherwise you'll be very dirty. It's like leaving the door to your home wide open for any stranger to enter, good or bad. If bad people enter, they will destroy you, hurt you, rob you, and fully mess things up. Samvar bhāvana is like closing the front door.

There are 18 kinds of sources of karma that can enter through your front door. Karma is a very big subject and I won't go into much detail in this book. We are working on a Karma book now so that you can really understand it. Keep an eye out for it.

One of the biggest sources of karma is *mithyatva*. Mithyatva is having "wrong vision or being on the wrong path instead of the right one." For example, in the United States, there is the Ku Klux Klan, which is a group of white supremacists, and they strongly believe only the white man is the best. They hate everyone else who is non-white. This is not correct vision and shows their full ignorance, but they strongly believe for themselves that the white man is the best.

If you go to small towns in states like Mississippi or other Deep South states and you start talking about Buddha or someone else, they will say, "Oh, no, only Jesus. Jesus is the only savior. If you don't believe in Jesus, you will go to hell." Their beliefs are so strong they cannot break the idea that there have been other spiritual teachers in the past, there are spiritual teachers presently, and there will be in the future. The word "only" is very dangerous. When you use the word "only" you exclude all possibilities. If Jesus taught unconditional love, and his followers today really understood and practiced unconditional love, then the word "only" cannot exist within their belief system. I don't blame followers of religions especially if they lacked education and heard one name over and over again. It is best to always be open-minded. There is always something to learn from somebody — take the good things, practice them and live them. Condemning others for not believing in what you do shows your ignorance more than the people you are trying to convert. All of this reflects mithyatva or lack of right vision.

When you stop the karma from entering into you, you begin to increase your right vision. When your karma that is blocking your vision begins to burn, then you begin to see truth as it really is. Not what you believe it to be or what it should be, but truth as it is. That's why samvar bhāvana is very important.

There are many religions in this world. I respect them all. Each of them has good ideas for society to help people keep calm. The important thing is that they follow and practice the good things. If one religion says, "Thou shall not kill. Thou shall not lie. Thou shall not steal" and teachings such as these, why are there millions of followers who kill (maybe not physically, but in their thoughts), why do they kill animals for food, why do they lie, why do they cheat people, why are they greedy and steal? But if people practiced the teachings wholeheartedly, then society will be a lot better. If you are a good person, you will automatically be a good Christian, Muslim, Buddhist, Hindu, Jain, or whatever you follow. But being Hindu, Muslim, Christian, or Jain doesn't automatically make you a good person. Many people say they follow and practice, and it could be more for show or to have a label or be part of a particular group, but in the end, it is best to be a good person, no matter what.

I see religions like different flowers in a garden. Many of them have a nice fragrance, but many flowers blossom without a fragrance. You have to be careful of the flowers that don't have a fragrance. There are religions which lack fragrance. Be careful. Otherwise it can lead you down the wrong path and bring you more sin and karma. Mithyatva brings a lot of karma to you.

When you are more spiritual than religious, you have a lot more potential for growth. You can then begin to stop the inflow of karma. You need to have the three jewels: *samyak darshan, samyak gnan, samyak charitrani moksh margah*. This means, "Right Vision, Right Knowing, and Right Conduct lead you to liberation." Living with these three jewels you automatically stop collecting karma because you are so aware that there are no chances of getting trapped into more karma.

The spiritual path which is given to you by an enlightened one can tell you how to improve yourself and how to live by those three jewels so that you can stop the inflow of karma. One specific teaching you can practice that will help you achieve these three jewels and help you live in samvar bhāvana is *Apramada*. Apramada means "always with awareness" and "no laziness." Even when you know what to do spiritually, it's very easy to become lazy. It's a lack of discipline and awareness. If you don't want to suffer, do something. When it's time for your practices, do them. Don't wait until tomorrow to do them. Do not leave things today for tomorrow. Tomorrow never comes. When you don't feel well, you still eat food and drink water, coffee or tea, right? Then why don't you do your spiritual practices? If you can't do an hour (if that's your usual), do 20 minutes. But still do it. If you allow your practices to slip, which is really the savior of your own path, then weakness increases and willpower decreases. Do something, even one mantra, once per day. This is better than nothing. Don't waste your life. Stop the inflow of karma.

Apramada was one of the last teachings of Tirthankara Mahavira, "Always be aware like a *bharand phaki*." A bharand phaki is a type of bird, which may be extinct now, and it has eyes which move in four directions. That bird is always alert. If you become alert like this bird, you are constantly in awareness. Awareness is not separate from you and it is actually effortless, you just need to keep burning your karma until you get there. It's better to be alert especially with your own inner negativities. It's interesting.

We worry about other people and can be mistrusting towards others, yet within you, you cannot even trust yourself to fight off your own inner enemies. You are worried about other people, but you have not mastered what is inside you. Be alert. As soon as negativity or anger comes, get rid of it somehow by shifting your thoughts to something positive or being grateful. Feel some kind of higher emotion to flow with.

Ultimately, you need to stop all good and bad karma. Good karma keeps you in the world longer, while bad karma makes you suffer. The longer your lives are, the more chances you have for falling backwards and getting trapped and collecting more bad karma. The best thing is to get out of it. Samvar bhāvana helps you to stop the inflow, but now you need to learn how to get rid of what is still remaining inside of you. You need to clean the house after all the damage has been done. That is Nirjara bhāvana.

9. Nirjara Bhāvana. *Nirjara* means "shedding of the karma particles." Continuing with the earlier example of cleaning your house: the door to your home was open and good and bad people entered your home ultimately destroying it and making it very dirty. You were finally able to close the door so that no one could enter, but you were still left with the mess they left behind. Nirjara bhāvana is the intention where you are always thinking to clean the mess up, to get rid of the karma. In the end, you are ultimately responsible and have to clean everything up. If you had vision, awareness, and strength, the front door would've always been closed.

There are two types of nirjara. One is called *akaam nirjara*, where the karmic particles shed or get cleaned naturally or without intention. These karmic particles go away on their own. Maybe they were light karmic particles so they didn't give much karmic result. The second is *sakaam nirjara* which is the intentional removal of the karma. There are several tools to help you to intentionally clean up your karma and that is through sadhana (spiritual practices), tapas (fasting), meditation, yoga, etc. The bhāvanas can help clean up the karmic mess. I always suggest for you to put effort.

In Indian mythology, there is a story about an angelic messenger named Narda who was very close to God. Narda loved to fly in the sky and was also fond of monks.

One day, he spotted two monks meditating in the forest and came down to visit them. He saw that there was an older monk doing his mala (rosary). The older monk asked, "Narda, are you going back to God?"

"Yes, I am going!"

"Can you ask God how many more lives I have?"

"Yes, of course!"

Before Narda left to ask God, he visited the other monk who was fairly new on the path and young. He was kind of lost in his own world, happy, dancing, enjoying the moment. "I'm going to ask God about your teacher, how about you?"

The young monk didn't respond and continued dancing.

Narda asked God and it replied, "When you return, you will see that the monks are sitting under different trees. Count the leaves on those trees each of them are under and that's how many lives will be left for them."

While Narda was speaking to God, a storm had happened down on earth. The wind blew the leaves around. The older monk was sitting under an almost leafless tree. Narda flew back down to earth and was so excited to tell the older monk that he had very few lives left (based on the number of leaves left on the tree). The old monk became very upset at the answer, "A few more lives left? I have worked so hard all of this time. God has no justice!" The old monk threw his rosary. "I cannot believe it!!"

Narda saw that the younger monk was sitting under a tree covered in millions of leaves. He felt bad for the young monk, but he shared with him what God revealed, "You have as many lives left as there are many leaves on this tree." The young monk replied, "Wow! Wow! God is so compassionate. I am so grateful. The fact that I will be liberated one day is the biggest blessing." The young monk went deep into his joy and meditation. He was dancing happily. Overjoyed that he will one day be liberated even after millions of lives.

Narda returned to God and was surprised to see that the young monk was already sitting next to God. "How did this happen? You said he had millions of lives left," Narda asked.

God said, "This young monk burned all of his karma very quickly. He went so deep and his intentions became so pure that he burned all of his karma and already liberated himself. It is not in my hands. He dissolved his mind quickly. Whatever karma he had left, he burned it all. Everything!"

When the power of intention becomes so pure, it becomes so powerful to burn all the karma away. The highest, purest intention can all of a sudden destroy one's karma. It does not take days, years, or lives to burn. It can burn even within a few hours, but it depends on the level of intention. The purest level of intention is needed in order for this sort of thing to happen. You have to be totally into it. Totally in tune with it fully and flowing like the young monk. We never know what intention is hidden inside of us, it is amazing. That's why I always remind students, nothing is impossible.

10. Lok Bhāvana. *Lok* means "universe." There are actually two components to the universe. Lok is the universe as we know it which contains six substances:

jivaastikaya, ajivaastikaya, dharmastikaya, adharmastikaya, akash, and kaal. Jiva is soul and *asti* means "existence" and *kaya* means "body." Even though the soul is shapeless, it still has shapeless particles. Only an enlightened soul or one with keval jnana can see the shapeless particles. Ajiva is non-soul; this makes up all the particles of the universe which are not alive. Ajiva is simply matter. Ajivaastikaya exists and has shape to it, but no soul. Dharmastikaya are the particles in the universe which allow movement to occur. Like water is for a fish to swim, dharmastikaya particles allow things in the universe to move. Adharmastikaya is the universal substance which allows something to stop. If those particles do not exist, things would continue to move and move and move. There is no stopping. Akaashtikaya is space. Lastly, there is kaal, which means time. Kaal is debatable. If you ask any Jain, they will say there are six substances of the universe including time; however, if you ask a Jain scholar they will argue that kaal, time, is not a substance. They don't say kaalastikaya; they say kaal. It shows, by the word, that time has no existence or particles, and that is true.

Jains will say Tirthankara Mahavira stated kaal is one of the six substances, but then one must ask how an enlightened master could say that kaal, time, is true, when he knows time does not exist. This sixth teaching, like many other teachings, was most likely created after Tirthankara Mahavira and they just put his name to it. Because they saw how time does affect existence in the sense we see a baby grow old, or something grow from short to tall, and without time you cannot differentiate these things. In my opinion, kaal is not a substance. Time does not exist. However, for the sake of share sharing the "six-substances" I'm sharing them here.

Now *alok*, is the other side of the universe which is basically empty space. Nothing can exist there at all except adharmastikaya, akash, and "kaal." At the edge of the physical universe where life and movement are on the other side is infinite empty space. Not even a star or single bacteria lives there. You can't even try to put a finger to cross over to the alok because there is a wall of "no movement particles."

When you are in the lok bhāvana intention, you begin to realize the wholeness of the universe. You see and know how vast and expanded it really is. When you have this knowledge, you begin to ask yourself, "Out of this whole universe and existence, where do I stand?" If there is a map of the entire universe, maybe a tiny dot can represent our earth, but you won't find yourself on the map. So the realization begins to arise, "Who am I? Why do I think I am so special on this earth? Compared to the bigger picture of the universe, I'm really nothing. Why do I have such a big ego? For what?" When you begin to see how little you are compared to the whole universe your ego begins to shrink and you become humble. When you are humble, you automatically become great. If you try to be great, it doesn't happen. When you are empty, you can fill yourself with the whole universe, but if you are full of yourself, the universe cannot enter you.

Crush and dissolve your ego. Yes, soul is great. Soul is all powerful. Soul is eternal, bodiless, shapeless, formless, all-knowing. Your soul is like that. So are all the infinite other souls in the universe. There is nothing special about you. Don't have that ego. Don't have that arrogance. It's not to say you should think low about yourself, either. Be confident. When you know your soul, you know everything. When you let go of everything, you receive everything.

Understanding the greatness and vastness of the universe reminds you to keep perspective. You think you have problems? Let's say a crisis happens on earth, like a virus spreads. In the bigger perspective of the universe, those problems are very small and remember, all problems are temporary and they will pass. Don't get caught up into these things. Learn to flow. Learn to be positive. Learn to live in the present moment.

You will move forward in life, free like a bird, when you live with this intention.

11. Bodhi Durlabh Bhāvana. *Bodhi durlabh bhāvana* is very important. *Bodhi* means "the source of knowledge." *Dhurlab* means "difficult." So, the real knowing is difficult to achieve. Your luckiest day will be when you achieve right knowing. Every living being has a lot of knowing. Even an ant has some level of knowing. Instinctively, they know where the food is and they will go to it. The knowing power is mostly revealed when someone is a human. The human body has a developed brain. Even though animals have 5 senses and some mind, they are unable to become enlightened because their mind is not fully developed. A fully developed mind has the ability to help you grow spiritually. That's why I like to remind everyone that you are very lucky. By having a human body you have a very big treasure in your hand. You need to use it properly and wisely. Don't abuse your body. Your body is one of your greatest instruments.

According to Damsan Pahud Sutra and Uttaraddhyan Sutra, there are four things which are difficult to achieve: *mānussatam, sui, saddha, samjammi ya viriyam.*

Human life, mānussatam, is difficult to achieve, as it takes millions of lives just to achieve human birth. But mānushyata, humanity, is even more difficult to achieve. Like there are people all around us, but many hearts are cold and lack a care for humanity in them. We need more humanness and that is the most difficult to achieve. Second, sui means "knowledge received from the teachings of an enlightened one" — Tirthankara or arihanta. You cannot get right knowing without sui. Jains interpret sui as one who "has heard that knowledge directly from a Tirthankara." This is a limited belief because anyone can listen to an enlightened one's teachings; it is not limited just to Tirthankaras. Fortunately, Jain scriptures contain 10% of truth, which is a lot for ancient text whereas most scriptures found in other religions have around 1% of truth.

I always suggest studying scriptures and with right guidance from a master you will have the deepest understanding of them — to know what is real and true and part of the 10% and know what is untrue. Sometimes teachings are based on an old society and that's why certain teachings require flexibility. Third, saddha is "right faith" but I interpret it more as "right vision." You need to attain right vision. No matter how much knowledge you have, without right vision, you may not go in the right direction. Lastly, samjammi ya viriyam, which means the strength for sadhana." You do the sadhana, but it's very difficult for you to follow it because you lack strength or you are not into it. In the Damsan Pahud Sutra, it states:

Damsanabhatthā bhatthā, damsanabhatthassa natthi nivvānam
Sijjhamti cariyabhatthā damsanabhatthā na sijjhamti

The person who has right vision is fully on the path. The people with no right vision cannot achieve liberation. The people who do not follow right behavior and have right conduct and habits still have chances to achieve liberation because they can again get back on the path. Their behavior, conduct, and way of thinking, talking and acting can change again, and their softness, bad conduct or character can progress again, but those who are polluted and far away from samyak darshan, or right vision, will never achieve liberation.

So, bodhi durlabh is very difficult to achieve. You cannot achieve bodhi without right vision. Once a person has right vision, they will automatically go in the right direction and the bodhi, then, will not be difficult to achieve.

When you have this bhāvana, intention, and think about how difficult it is to achieve the knowing, you will push yourself to follow mānussatam, sui, saddha, and samjammi ya viriyam. Achieving human life with humanness, getting in touch with an enlightened one's teachings, having right vision, and gaining strength to do your spiritual practices. These four things are difficult to achieve, but when you get it, the *sambodhi* is not far. Sambodhi means "total knowing."

Most people have indirect knowledge. Indirect knowledge is when you read a book, learn from a teacher, watch something on TV or on the internet, or hear something from someone else. That knowledge came from an external source. When knowledge comes externally, then that is not soul knowledge. A person who is a scholar and can quote all spiritual things can be mesmerizing, but it doesn't necessarily mean they are in touch with direct knowledge — soul knowledge. Indirect knowledge is not difficult to achieve, but direct knowledge from the soul is the most difficult to achieve. That is why it is so precious once it is attained.

Those who are born into the Jain religion sometimes have a big ego about it. They think, "We have the best karma, we are born as Jains, we have the knowledge of the Tirthankaras," and so on. They're merely entertaining themselves. If one is a Jain and then go out and gamble, eat meat, drink alcohol, go to prostitutes, or do a lot of bad things, then how are they special? There's no spirituality in those things. There's no growth. That is not living and practicing the Tirthankaras' teachings. When you are not born Jain, and you are on the spiritual path, you are living and practicing non-violence to the best of your abilities, you try and learn and practice sadhana, and your karma is like a Jain, then that is the best thing. Jain means the followers of the enlightened ones - the Jinas - who have victory over themselves. In reality, the Jain system shouldn't be considered a religion, but a way of life.

An enlightened person's teachings have no boundaries. They don't create religions or sects. Spiritual teachings are universal. All living beings can enjoy and benefit from them. So for Jains to think they are the *only* ones to have access to the Tirthankaras' teachings, then it only shows ego. They also believe that no enlightened masters exist after the last Tirthankara Mahavira - no arihantas and no liberation. It is too bad. If they can experience direct knowing from their soul, they will know the reality. Most live with indirect knowledge without right vision.

The best thing is to have direct knowledge from your soul. Purify your mind. Purify your bhāvanas. It is the most difficult, but brings the greatest reward when achieved.

*12. **Dharma Bhāvana.*** *Dharma* means "the path." When

you live in the highest state of intention, then you've attained the real path. The real path is what sets your soul free. In the end, you have to let go of all the beliefs you've ever had and begin to realize the truth. This aspect is not easy because you are like shedding those parts of yourself. The culture, religion, society and family you grew up in gave you your mind. Dissolving your mind is the highest and most difficult form of surrender. It is the heavy mind, dravya manas, that keeps you away from your soul, yet you need the developed and higher/ spiritual mind, bhāva manas, to get you close to your soul. In the end, you leave your mind behind. This is living the real path. This is living in soul.

To help you live on the right path, you surrender to these five special types of souls: arihantas (enlightened ones), *siddhas* (liberated souls or God in pure bodiless form), *acharyas* (spiritual leaders), *upadhyayas* (spiritual teachers — the real ones), and *sadhu/sadhvis* (monks/nuns). Surrender to them and seek their company. When you surrender, you are open to guidance. There is no ego. When there is no ego, there is no resistance to their suggestions. It's the ego and lower mind which fights truth. Ego wants to rule. It doesn't want to die. That's why in a way, you must die before you die. When you surrender, your mind is dead and you can receive the right guidance to grow. Keep the company of these five types of souls.

It's difficult to find the real ones, but they are there out in the world. The truth seeker won't give up to find them, to learn from them, and they will put all the effort to meet them. Truth seekers are so thirsty, and when you're thirsty for truth, you'll do everything you can to find the real water. Be aware of the company you keep. If you live with negative people, you will naturally become negative. If you live with toxic people, you will feel like you can't breathe and feel so heavy. If you live with friends or have friendship with those who drink alcohol and do drugs, you'll most likely do the same thing. If you're friends with monks and spiritual teachers, can you really go backwards on the path? If you have the chance or opportunity to be connected with these five souls, you will begin to break all of your ideas and begin to live a pure life.

When you live with these 12 bhāvanas, you will live closely to your soul. Your bhāva manas will reflect who you really are. You will see and know your soul.

3 | How To Purify Your Intentions

When you practice the 12 bhāvanas (intentions or reflections), you will begin to see a shift in your life. Here are 10 practical ways you can improve your intentions:

MAITRI BHĀVANA

In the Jain system, which I consider more a way of life for every living being versus a religion, they teach additional intentions which can be practiced especially by non-monks. The reason they are not included in the twelve is because they serve more as tools than intentions. These four bhāvanas are more like virtues and qualities versus state of mind and consciousness. They can be practiced.

A beautiful quality to have is *maitri*, which means "friendship." If there is no friendship with others, then animosity or enmity builds. The most important friendship is the one you have with yourself. You need to live, think highly of yourself, love and care for yourself. When you have friendship with yourself, then you can share that friendship with other people because you have developed this quality. When you have something, you can spread or share it.

Friendship is a uniting force - whether it is between two people or many people. There is a unity. If there is no friendship, there is no unity. One day, as you grow on the spiritual path, you will extend your friendship to all living beings. If you are friends with all living beings, can you hurt them? Kill them? Hate them? Be mean to them? First, you need to master friendship with yourself. When you develop this and begin to connect with other living beings, then you become like a mother to them. You have a special connection, a special friendship, like a mother has with her own baby.

Maitri Bhāvana is needed to help you grow spiritually higher because when this quality is developed automatically your intentions become pure. But without friendship, you cannot grow further. Friendship brings relaxation to you, not stress. If there is no friendship with yourself, you will always be disturbed. If you are not friendly with other living beings, you will be disturbed and affected. If you approach an animal and you are not friendly or relaxed, the animal will sense your fear or uncomfortableness, then out of their own fear and need to survive, they might bite or hurt you. When there is friendship with all living beings, there is no reaction, there is no fear.

One special sutra that we as monks recite every day from the Pratikraman sutra is:

Khamemi savve jiva
savve jiva khamantu me
mitti me savva bhuyesu
veram majha na kenai

I forgive all living beings.
May all living beings grant me forgiveness.
My friendship is with all living beings.
I have no enmity towards any living being.

When you are friends with yourself and all living beings, you have no enemies. That is where freedom is. You have nothing to fear. There is a common saying that "You are your own worst enemy." People are enemies to themselves and that's why they are unhappy, unfree, depressed. When you unconditionally love yourself and others, know how to forgive yourself and others, then life will be totally different for you. Your state of mind will be higher and higher. It's the higher state of mind that helps you grow.

The maitri bhāvana eases you totally. People come to Siddhayatan Tirth & Retreat (Texas) to take workshops on how to relieve stress and tension. One of the first lessons I share is the need to be friendly with yourself. Without such friendship, the stress and tension will always remain. It's an important quality and virtue to develop. You begin to feel that "oneness with all living beings," which is non-violence. You feel, "I am alive, they are alive. I feel pain, they feel pain. I get hurt, they get hurt. There is no difference between me and them." This is non-violence, this is friendship, this is freedom.

Maitri plays a big role in your life. It creates friendliness in you. Friendliness is your intention. Understandably, everyone's on different levels of spiritual path and understanding and not everyone will be friends. It is not expected. What you can control is your higher thinking and your own friendliness. Be wise with your friendships, also. You need to be smart. One tip I can share with you is not to tell your friends everything. Don't share all your secrets. Be careful, because those same family or friends can hurt you and use those things as weapons. When you are aware of what you keep to yourself, then you will have no fear of others hurting you with your own words. You cannot control others and you must protect yourself, but you have to be the smart and wise one not to say anything.

PRAMOD BHĀVANA

Pramod Bhāvana is another important quality or virtue to develop. *Mod* means "happiness" and *pramod* means "a lot of happiness." If you learn to be happy with yourself, then you can be happy with others. Most people are not happy with themselves and blame others for their unhappiness. Pramod really connects with the happiness experienced from learning to appreciate others.

Happiness cannot exist without appreciation, and appreciation is required to develop this bhāvana. When we appreciate others, we automatically respect them, honor them, and reduce jealousy or negative feelings towards them. If you are ever feeling down, think about something you are grateful for - within yourself or from others. Gratitude and appreciation lift the spirit high. Life is not long, time passes by quickly, so it is better to be in happiness and live with appreciation.

When you think of others, think positively of them. Celebrate their successes. Speak highly of them. Lift people up. Be genuinely happy for other people's happiness. Oftentimes, people are jealous of others. Jealousy brings you down. If you are satisfied and content with your life, there is no room for jealousy. Think highly, spread the happiness and appreciation, and others will be inspired by your happiness.

Appreciate whoever you live with or whoever you meet. Find something good in them and appreciate it. If you have a pet, love your bird, give affection to your dog, cat, hamster or even pet cow. All living beings enjoy appreciation, affection, and care. You will automatically feel good when you live in this state of being; most importantly, you will have peace.

KARUNA BHĀVANA

Karuna Bhāvana is "compassion" and it can destroy all of your karma. Compassion increases a lot of qualities inside of a person. Out of pain or feeling sympathy or concern, you try and help. For example, a mother is very compassionate towards her child. If the child gets hurt, she feels the hurt. This is because she is connected to the child and considers them a part of her. When you feel the same, when you feel another person or animal or any other living being is a part of you, and not separate from you, you will also feel the pain. Sometimes there is too much pain you feel and you will do everything you can to help.

There are three main types of pain: physical, mental, and spiritual. When you are compassionate, you begin to free yourself of your own pain. It may seem selfish, but the reality is, the pain you experience when you see someone or something get hurt is your own pain. Whatever the other is going through is merely a cause or trigger to the pain you already have inside of you. Everyone has pain. And, when we help others, not only are we relieving our own pain, but can help reduce someone else's pain too. That's how compassion burns your karma; you're inspired to help others and yourself, which burns your karma and pain.

There are many ways to help others depending on the situation. Maybe taking care of someone who is sick, donating to a cause you care about, or listening to someone so that they can vent. There are many ways. People feel they can't help, or their help isn't enough. Some problems in the world seem so big, you might think, "Well, what can I do?" You can always do something. Even helping one person or one soul changes their life. Thinking positively is a very big help especially when crisis happens or natural disasters happen. We need more positivity than negativity and fear. If you're unable to donate, donate a little bit; everything really helps and adds up for the non-profit organizations so they can help. However, you can also help by inspiring others to give, if you're unable to give yourself. Remember, it's all about your intention. All efforts count out of your compassion. Never forget that.

As you begin to feel oneness with all living beings and compassion for all, the time comes you become or feel like a mother to all living beings. Compassion is one of the best qualities to develop in your life.

Consider this perspective: Teaching compassion is more important than teaching charity. Compassion is a quality that lasts forever and will affect all areas of your life and help others. Whereas, if you feed the poor only once, out of charity, that help is limited - that compassion is limited. But, if someone learns to be compassionate, they will always be compassionate, their help is never-ending in small or big ways. We need more compassionate people, then you will see everything will begin to shift around you and around the world.

MADHYASTA BHĀVANA

Madhyasta Bhāvana is the greatest quality, which is "being neutral." Whether people praise you or criticize you, you remain the same. You are unaffected. You don't take sides. When you are neutral, no matter what is happening, you will not collect karma, because there is no reaction.

The truth is: Madhyasta is the shortest path towards liberation. It's not easy at all, but if you master it, it is the best thing because you stop collecting karma and begin to burn it quickly.

Here's an example of being neutral. A nanny is taking care of the baby. She feeds the baby, cleans the baby, looks after the baby, and does the very best she can while the baby is in her care. Deep down, she knows that this baby is not hers, even though she is doing more than the mother. This is known as being neutral. She still serves. If we become neutral, like this nanny, this is achieving madhyasta bhāvana. The nanny will not cry once the care-taking job is over because she always knew that child was never hers.

Or, if there is a good judge, an uncorrupted judge, they will hear both sides of the case neutrally. Their intent is not to destroy the defendant, hurt them, their family, etc. The judge listens, considers the best ruling, which is fair and just. There is a lot of gossip and rumor that happens on the media or even among family members. If you get affected by gossip or show an interest in it, you are not practicing being neutral. There are always two sides to the story and then there is the absolute Truth. If you react to gossip and are taken by it, then you are far away from being neutral and balanced. It's like you take pleasure in hearing or reading the stories or enjoy hearing someone else's misery. It's best not to take sides. Don't make any judgments. Hear both sides first before coming to your own conclusion. A one-sided story is incomplete. Hearing the other side can bring more understanding and clarity. Be a higher person, not a lower-quality person.

PRANAYAMA

Pranayama is one of the best systems to control and discipline your senses and mind. Pranayama means "controlling your pranic force." Some call it "breath work." Pranayama helps with purifying your senses and removing the toxins in your body, especially your nervous system, respiratory system, endocrine system, and organs. If toxins are built up in your body, then your instrument is not pure. If your instrument is not pure, it can send the wrong messages to your mind. Pranayama is part of the yogic system which helps you to relax, loosen, and lighten your whole body, senses, and mind.

You need a light body to progress spiritually. I'm not referring to your body weight. Your subtle bodies need to be light. When you are light, you float, you flow, and spiritually you go upwards. If you are full of heaviness and lots of toxins, you will be with negative thoughts, be depressed and anxious, and never happy. How can you have high intentions if you are heavy inside? The lighter you become, the purer you are. When you have a light body, light nerves, light senses and nothing is hidden, there is nothing to corrupt you or stop you from being close to the soul.

We think it's easy to access soul through meditation. And most people try guided meditation and maybe they feel some peace, but mostly they cannot access the deepest part of them — the real meditation. In order to really be in meditation, you have to have a light body; a light body won't have tension or stress (which prevents meditation), a person will be a vegetarian, as meat creates heaviness and brings a lot of toxins to the body, and when someone is light you don't even have to try and meditate because it just happens. But what do people do? I've seen it. So-called meditation teachers and yogis (even some monks!) will eat meat, drink alcohol, and do ayahuasca — these are the worst things and they make your inner body heavier not lighter. These people lack vision. That's why it is important to seek right guidance. Oftentimes, the blind leads the blind. If anyone encourages you or says it's ok to put these heavy toxins into your body (beef, pork, chicken, fish, alcohol, drugs, ayahuasca, etc.) then I suggest you stay far away from them. They will not lead you to your soul because they themselves are far away from their soul.

It's interesting to know that people drink alcohol to relax, but when they drink they get violent or go crazy, so how is that real relaxation? When a person becomes an alcoholic or drug addicted, it's even harder to bring out what is buried inside. That's why it's best to not even do those things.

There are many pranayama techniques; however, I will share with you three simple pranayama techniques that you can do to help clear your senses, nervous system, and brain. You will begin to feel lighter and less tensed. The first one is *anulom vilom*. Anulom vilom is "alternative nostril breathing." The way I describe and teach it is considered untraditional. The traditional one is not as powerful as this way. Anulom vilom helps clear your sun and moon channels. There are three main channels in your body. The sun channel (*pingala*) which is on the right side, the moon channel (*ida*) which is on the left, and the third channel (*sushumna*) which is up and down your spine. When you do anulom vilom your nerves begin to relax. The emotions like anger, ego, greediness, jealousy, negativities, low self-esteem, etc. will be released, and you will begin to feel light. Remember, we want to remove any pollution or corruption that blocks you from having a pure dravya manas and bhāva manas.

For anulom vilom, take your right hand and place your right ring finger and press down on your left nostril. Breathe in very slowly yet intensely through the right nostril. When it is time to exhale, switch and close off your right nostril with your right thumb and exhale out slowly and steadily until all air is expelled through the left nostril. Don't hold your breath, continue breathing, and switch back and forth. Basically, the right ring finger closes the left nostril, inhale, then switch closing off the right nostril with your right thumb and exhale out. Do this for three minutes daily. If you can do more, do more. The best time to practice anulom vilom is early in the morning when there is more oxygen outside.

The next technique is a four-step breathing combination I created. You need to be sitting down, whether in a chair or cross-legged, with your spine relaxed and straight. Then tilt your head back looking up towards the ceiling and exhale forcefully through your nose with your belly going in while keeping your mouth closed. Your inhale will happen automatically and quickly. Then look all the way down, almost as if your chin is to your chest, then exhale out forcefully through your nose. Inhale automatically. Bring your head back to neutral then turn your head left, exhaling out (inhale is automatic), then turn your head right, exhaling out (inhaling automatically right after). Keep doing this repetition: up, down, left, right exhaling out every time. Mouth closed, forceful exhalation through your nose. Basically, you're doing the *kapalbhati* breath in combination with the different positions of your head. Do this set for at least three minutes. You will feel your senses becoming light. You might feel light-headed, spacy or dizzy. Try your best to really force out all the air in the exhalation. The more forceful it is, the more you are able to release those stubborn toxins that are in your body. This exercise will help release the stress in your shoulders, neck, and head. If you have severe neck issues, avoid doing this practice.

The third pranayama technique is *nadi shodhan* which means "nerve purification." This is an excellent technique to remove the tension from your nervous system. If your nerves are not well it brings a lot of tension, stress, nervousness, worry, and anxiety to you. If your nerves are not relaxed, how can they pass on the right message to your brain and mansa? That's why it's very important to clear your senses and nerves with the breathing techniques I'm sharing with you.

For nadi shodhan, you first need to take your right hand and close off your left nostril with your right ring finger. Keeping your mouth closed, exhale out of your right nostril twice. On each exhale your belly goes in. You will then have an automatic inhale in between each exhale. Then close off your right nostril with your right thumb and exhale out twice. Keep going back and forth with this breathing technique for at least three minutes. You will feel all of your nerves, which are in the millions, begin to clear. Actually, there are 72,000 main nerves in the body. With this breathing technique, you will begin to clear all of them. These nerves are what bring you and keep you in illusion and confusion. With these two things, your mind will constantly be in a mess and far from your soul. These breathing techniques will also help you if you practice them right before you meditate.

As a result of doing pranayama, you will be releasing a lot of things that are very much compressed in your body. Don't be surprised that if after some time of doing these breathing exercises, your emotions begin to come up on the surface. They will show themselves. You might cry, you might be angry, you might experience pain, and you will not know where it is coming from. Rest assured and understand that whatever was hidden underneath and the things you may have forgotten will come up. If they don't come out of you, they will always control you or affect you. Eventually, you'll reach a point that your body, senses, and mind are so crystal clear; you will finally feel free. This is the whole point of spirituality. It's a process. It takes time. It takes practice. It takes discipline. It takes perseverance. Never give up and one day you will reach your goal.

Many years ago, I was in New Delhi and a group of 10

friends came to visit me at night for advice. The friends had a kind of bet with each other going on. One of the friends knew 15 languages, but because he was so intelligent and mastered each language, none of the friends knew what his original language was. The linguistic friend challenged the rest of the friends that if they guessed his original language he would give them 15,000 rupees. They all tried and failed. India has many languages and dialects, and their challenge was to guess the right one. So they asked me to help so that they can win. It was all for fun.

I said I could help them guess with one condition. They would need to spend the night at the ashram and keep their door open. I told them between the evening and morning they will discover what the original language is. It was summer, so they were able to sleep on the carpeted floor with their pillows. They kept talking past midnight. I was keeping an eye on the main guy to make sure he was fully asleep. When he fell into a deep sleep, I slapped him in a way that it made a loud sound. He called me a bad name in his original language. Because when you are fast asleep and something shocks you, you will react in your own language.

In the morning, I told all the friends and he confirmed I was right. I said "give that money to the poor people, I don't need it." Why I share this story is because your senses, nerves, and mind are in a deep sleep and you have to shake them and hit them badly so that you can wake up. Pranayama helps wake those sleeping idiots (senses, mind, brain,, nervous system, etc.) up. Intensive breathing wakes them up even quicker.

Unless you purify your body and mind, you cannot go deep into your bhāva manas. Bhāva manas is not catchable or visible. It is a reflection of the soul, as it is the closest part of mind to your soul. It is not touchable, but you can try to understand it. To do so, you must purify yourself. A purified intention is the most powerful.

PRESENT MOMENT LIVING

You only exist in the present moment. You can be in-tune with your soul in the present moment. When you are in your mind, you are disconnected from your soul and mostly live in the past or future. Both cause depression or anxiety respectively. Learning to be present teaches you how to be aware in every moment. A simple technique is to test yourself throughout the day - *Am I with soul? Am I with my mind? Where are my thoughts? What is my body feeling? What are my senses experiencing?* In general, these are some way to live in the present moment and to check in. When you are present, you are engaged. Your mind is not wandering off. You are on duty. You are able to learn, absorb, understand. If your mind is in worry, guilt, fear, repeating memories, reliving something in your mind, or being in desires, imagination and fantasy, then you are not living in the present moment. You're in illusion.

The teaching to live in the present moment is not a new thing. Learning to be aware is not a new thing. Learning to be "in the now" is not new. These teachings are all ancient and have been practiced for thousands, if not millions of years. The Tirthankaras, the enlightened ones, always taught about awareness. When you are present, when you are on duty, when you are aware, you will observe and be a witness to your thoughts, actions, and speech. When you are in this space, you are likely to collect less karma or even prevent yourself from collecting karma.

In western countries, a lot of people wear the cross as

Jesus was crucified on the cross. It is a very popular symbol in Christianity, but interestingly enough people do not understand the deep symbolism behind it. You have two lines: One moves horizontally (the shorter line), and the other moves vertically (the longer line). This symbol actually comes from the Shramanic tradition.

The long line represents your soul. As the soul awakens, it moves upwards towards enlightenment and liberation. The shorter line, which moves horizontally, is your mind which goes between the past and the future. When you live in the mind, it keeps you in the world of suffering. It goes back and forth, back and forth like waves of the ocean always splashing around. There's no peace when you live in the mind.

When you live in the present moment, you are automatically living in the vertical line. Now, you have to work hard on yourself to move upwards towards liberation. It's not easy, but it is worth it in the end. There is so much power in soul. We think the mind is quick. We think using the brain at the 100% level is powerful. Imagine how fast and powerful the soul is. The mind is nothing compared to the soul.

I can guarantee that if someone gets enlightened and they are leaving their body at that moment, the soul will reach the highest point of the universe before their body hits the floor. The highest point of the universe, where all the liberated souls reside, is called *siddhaaloka*. It is located at the boundaries of the universe (loka) before the aloka (where nothing exists except space). Soul has so much speed and power. The mind cannot compete with the soul, nor can it comprehend it. Instead of feeding your mind, feed your soul. Wake up.

Purify your mind so that you can become mindless. Dissolve your mind and you'll enter the mindless state. When you close off your senses and disconnect from your mind in a relaxed way, you can begin to taste soul in meditation. That is the real meditation. Anytime you force meditation, you are in the mind. Relax. Let go. Move vertical.

Understand deeply that there is no past and there is no future. It is all an illusion. Yesterday is gone. It is never going to come back to you. So why bother wasting your time thinking about yesterday? And tomorrow never comes because it is always today. If a person understands that it is always today, then that is how they can live in the present moment.

The breathing techniques I mentioned before will help you to live in the present moment. Specifically anulom vilom or nadi shodhan. When your body is clear, your body is free of toxins; you don't even have to try to live in the present moment. You are already living it.

FASTING

One of the best steps to help you grow, purify your body and mind is the practice of *tapas* — fasting. This helps you to practice nirjara bhāvana. There are two types of tapas: internal fasting *(āntrik tapa)* and external fasting *(bāhya tapa)*. Fasting means to abstain and have the discipline to stay away from something. Your senses are out of control. When your senses are out of control, then so is your mind. When you give into cravings or what your senses really like or give into desires of the mind, you lose control over yourself. When you crave something, you begin to create addiction. Your soul loses all power when your senses and mind are just feeding you useless things — out of fun, good taste, or something else.

On the spiritual path, you need to have discipline, willpower, and self-control. Even when you control yourself a little bit than you normally would, that is more helpful versus nothing at all. Fasting is a very big and important practice. I published a water fasting book that goes over everything in more detail so you can understand and practice it.

For the purpose of living with higher intention, I suggest to start fasting and give your body a little break. There are many types of fasts that you can do. Here are some examples. You can water fast, which means you only drink water. You can do a dry fast, which means you have no food or water. I would not suggest doing a dry fast more than 24 hours if you are not experienced. You can practice *unodri*, which means "eating less than what you are hungry for." For example, if you know you are hungry for two pieces of bread, you eat only one. You can eat only one meal per day, which is called *ekasna*. Or, beasna which means eating twice a day. Anything you do with a limit is considered fasting.

These days, intermittent fasting is becoming quite popular. But this practice is nothing new or revolutionary; however, it is highly being marketed as such. Intermittent fasting is good. I'm not putting it down; however, it's best not to live in illusion as if this is a new discovery. People have been fasting for millions of years to cleanse their body for spiritual growth and upliftment. Fasting is part of the Shramanic tradition and many monks and people around the world practice fasting for spiritual reasons today. Fasting is good for your health and it helps you burn a lot of karma.

Every year, millions of people around the world celebrate *Paryushan* - the celebration of soul - which is usually in August or September. Spiritual practitioners fast for the 8-day celebration or if they are unable to fast all 8 days, they will alternate, and if they don't do that, they all will fast on the last day of celebration. Can you imagine what happens to the world when millions of people are fasting together, are in a positive mood, and are in non-violence? It brings so much positive energy to the world to help balance out the negativity. Never think a small group of people can't make a difference.

When a person fasts, they immediately create willpower, they have control and discipline over their senses, and a fire is created within them to burn the toxins in their body and the karma that surrounds the soul. It's not an easy practice. For some people it can be easy depending on their body and for some it could be a very torturing experience, maybe because their body has too much acidity in it. Consider fasting at least one day, this month, for 24 hours drinking only water. Try it. It will be the most beneficial to you, your body, mind and soul.

MANTRAS

Mantras are divine sounds that when repeated aloud or in your mind (*japa*) they create a lot of higher energy for you. They help your health, mind, and learning abilities, protect you, and help to raise your consciousness. The power of a mantra helps not only by reciting, but by feeling it too. Be in tune with it and do the mantra whole-heartedly. There are so many mantras out there that are used for different reasons. For your spiritual growth and advancement, I suggest you master the *Namokar* mantra. The Namokar mantra is a universal mantra that can help you in so many ways. There is a big science to the Namokar mantra that one book can be dedicated to it; however, for the power of raising your intentions, raising your energy and uplifting your soul, learning to pronounce and doing the mantra every day will help you a lot.

The Namokar mantra teaches you to be humble and to take refuge in the five special souls in this universe. This mantra helps you to automatically crush your ego because this is considered a "bowing down" mantra. *Namo* means "I bow." This mantra will help you attain right knowledge and overcome the difficulties as mentioned with the bodhi durlabh bhāvana.

Namo Arihantānam
Namo Siddhānam
Namo Aiyariyānam
Namo Uvajjhayānam
Namo Loe Savva Sahunām

Eso Pancha Namokaro
Savva Pavvapanasano
Mangala Nam Cha Savvesim
Padhāmam Havai Mangalam

If you take refuge with the Arihanta, your knowing

power will increase because the Arihanta is the best guide to show you the path, to teach you about spirituality and the best way to burn your own karma. They are enlightened souls with a last body so they are still able to communicate with you unlike God/Siddha. Secondly, take refuge in God, or *siddha*, the liberated souls. Pay respect to them, connect to them, be inspired by them. They have liberated themselves and so can you. When you surrender totally to God, your mind must disappear. It is the most freeing. Your ego will totally be gone. Take refuge in the *Acharyas* or spiritual leaders. They are already on the right path and can guide you to increase your bhāvana to become purer and purer. If you can find an *Upadhyaya*, or spiritual teacher, then take shelter and refuge in them, they will guide you and help you get rid of all your wrong vision, ignorance and illusion which keeps you roaming in this world of suffering.

Surrender to the renunciants — the monks and nuns — as they are on the right and true path. When you have friendship with them, they can help you in your spiritual journey and advise you how to practically advance and grow. This mantra is all about surrender, taking refuge, paying respect, and honoring the advancement of these great souls. It is through these souls that the path is continued to be shared and made practical. These are the real spiritual teachers and guides. Learn as much as you can from them.

What's amazing with this mantra is that it is written in plural form. There is not just one enlightened person, one liberated soul, one best spiritual leader, or one best spiritual teacher or one best monk or nun. When you recite this mantra you are bowing down infinite times to all of these souls that are throughout the universe. Can you imagine the power when you recite this mantra more than once? It's like bowing down infinite and infinite times. Over and over again. When you really get into it and feel it within you and connect to them, your energy will be so high and you will feel incredibly light and your heart totally open. This is a beautiful mantra to really help you with you reaching the higher states of consciousness and intention. If you can, try to practice this mantra at least 27 or 108 times per day. It'll take some time to get used to pronouncing it and memorizing it correctly, but be patient. Do the practice. It will help you a lot.

SELF-ANALYSIS

A very important step is self-analysis. When you begin to analyze yourself, you will be surprised: your negativity will disappear and your pure intention appears. I suggest for you to get a dedicated journal for self-analysis then find a private place in your home where you can be. For 30 minutes, reflect about all the mistakes you've made during the day since the morning up until the time you sat down. Try recalling if you yelled at someone, or maybe suppressed your anger, maybe you said bad words, or you killed a spider. Maybe you hit someone or maybe you lied. Write down every mistake you can think of that you did with your actions, thoughts and speech, and even note your impure intentions — knowingly or unknowingly. Sometimes you are in a good mood, so there's maybe less on that day or if you're in a bad mood you might have more. Whatever you remember, write it down in your journal. Do this technique every day. You might end up with 30-40 lines per day.

Then after a week begin to compare your notes. See what similar themes and mistakes are happening each day. When you become aware of what you are doing, the less you will do it. You will cringe and not be happy with your mistakes so you'll want to change them. By paying attention to your bad habits and mistakes, they will begin to reduce. It's like a shy monster. The monster is scary, but as soon as you start to pay attention it loses its power.

Self-analysis is a form of criticizing yourself, but for good reason. Consider it "constructive criticism." Without identifying your weaknesses in detail you will not be able to improve them. Identifying your mistakes is a big thing because it also takes courage to face yourself and to admit your mistakes. It creates humility within yourself too. It's easy to criticize others. Instead we should see our shortcomings first and then you'll less likely be so hard on others. Become aware of your mistakes and compare your actions day-to-day and your negative thoughts will begin to disappear.

You need to stare at your weaknesses, mistakes, and negativity. When you stare at them, they become uncomfortable and then embarrassing. This is how to reduce their power over you. This is how to increase your level of intentions. After a week or two weeks of practice, you will become better and better each day and being aware during the day and remembering your mistakes. The time will come where your list will become shorter and shorter. Sometimes on the spiritual path it's difficult to feel like you're progressing. When you record things, you will see your progress. That's why journaling helps. Make sure to keep your journal in a safe and secure location where no one can see it. Remember, what I shared with you before: Never share your deepest secrets with others. Those secrets become weapons when a relationship goes sour or becomes unsteady. You cannot trust people with your secrets. Keep things to yourself. Not everything is everyone's business.

Self-analysis is a great tool to help you get out of this pollution. The biggest pollution in the whole universe are everyone's thoughts. Smoke is not the biggest pollution. Our thoughts, especially the negative ones, are the greatest pollution in the universe. Real climate change begins with changing one's thoughts. Thoughts can make you suffer a lot and make your life miserable. It makes others suffer too. It's better to be away from them and be with your soul.

The best thing to achieve and realize is the state of

blankness, nothingness, or enlightenment. Enlightenment is blank! No thoughts at all! And that kind of blankness is something super, special and extraordinary. Purify your thoughts and automatically your mind becomes pure. When your mind is pure, you will begin to think purely, and everything you do is with pure intention.

DIRECT GUIDANCE

One of the most important steps to help you reach your spiritual goals and help you connect to your soul is to have right guidance. You can have all of the tools, all of the books, and a lot of experience, but without right guidance you can still go backwards on your journey. Having right guidance, in a way, is your safety net. If you are able to learn from an *arhat*, or enlightened one, who has already purified their intention and lives in soul, then that is the best person who can guide you. They have gone through the journey. When you listen and practice their advice, it is the biggest boost for your path. The key thing is to not only have the right guide, but to practice what they are suggesting to you as well. Monks and nuns of the spiritual path can be helpful for you too. They have gone through the experiences. They have also worked hard on themselves. They may be close to enlightenment so they can guide you along the way. They have very deep meditation experiences and know the soul. They may just have a little karma left, but those little karmas won't deter them. They have purified their intention. Seek guidance from those who realized it and have experienced it. If they have reached a pure state of intention, you are in good hands.

Direct guidance means receiving guidance from those who know what renunciation is. There are many people out in the world who are happy to give out advice. They will outline all the steps for you to become enlightened, or guarantee it, and even provide you with a certificate of enlightenment. There are a lot of motivational speakers, inspirational speakers, and best-selling authors, and in some ways it is good they share their journey and advice, but if they have not renounced the world, if they are still into the luxuries, if they are too much into their family, then they haven't understood what it means to live with pure intention. If they are too much into the world, providing inspirations on how to best live in the world and to attain worldly success, then how can they help you reach your high spiritual goals? Are you trying to be someone great in society? Or are you trying to liberate your soul? Answer this question honestly, and then you'll know which direction you will head. Ultimately, you do have to choose. You cannot have your feet in two boats. You have to choose — worldly life or spirituality.

When you choose spirituality, it doesn't mean you stop living in the world. Your life is actually still the same. You have to work. You have to pay the bills. You have your responsibilities, but the difference is the intention. When there is a shift within you that everything is about spirituality for you, then you are moving towards your inner freedom. Any challenges you go through, you overcome because you have a deeper understanding. Maybe it's karma. Maybe there's a lesson. Maybe you need to be more confident. When you are only about the world, then you suffer. Even if you have a lot of money, you won't have peace. And, if you're trying to use spirituality to help you achieve worldly goals, and have just enough spirituality to keep you a little positive, you're still not safe and you will still suffer. Once you renounce the world, the world cannot hurt you anymore. You know that the world is meaningless. Yes, you still do something with your life. Yes, you still help others. But there is no expectation of reward. You help because you want to help. You know your time on earth is temporary, so why not do something special for others and yourself?

That's why you need to seek guidance from those who already live their life that way. Learn from those who have renounced the world. Learn from those who are in the spiritual boat 100%, not the ones who are using spirituality to attract followers or gain fame and success. Seek the ones who are helping others wholeheartedly. They may not have a lot of students, and that's ok. A master doesn't need followers or students. The students need the master. A master, monk, or nun, they are happy alone — remember ekaatva bhāvana? They are complete within themselves. They don't really need anything. Just food, water, and some shelter to survive. Learn from them. They may have already achieved the inner peace and joy you are desperately seeking.

Social media, reading books, or watching videos of an enlightened one, monks, and nuns are very helpful, but you will still be missing one piece. You will miss out on the direct experience of feeling the presence of that soul. You won't be able to fully feel their energy. You will miss out on really seeing them, hearing them, and being close to them. Seek direct guidance. Make an effort to meet them. It can be the biggest blessing for your path. Remember, time runs faster than anything. Don't wait to meet the master. Receive guidance while they are alive. Eventually, their time on earth is over too. It's not too late, yet.

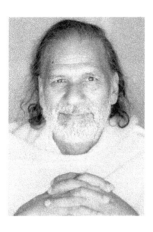

Acharya Shree Yogeesh is a living enlightened master of this era and is the founder of the Siddhayatan Tirth and Spiritual Retreat, a unique 250+ acre spiritual pilgrimage site and meditation park in North America providing the perfect atmosphere for spiritual learning, community, and soul awakening to help truth seekers advance spiritually. Acharya Shree is also the founder of the Yogeesh Ashram near Los Angeles, California, Yogeesh Ashram International in New Delhi, India, the Acharya Yogeesh Primary & Higher Secondary children's school in Haryana, India, and his latest establishment, Siddhayatan Mandir Estonia, in Eastern Europe.

As an inspiring revolutionary spiritual leader and in-demand speaker worldwide, for nearly fifty years Acharya Shree has dedicated his life to helping guide hundreds of thousands of people on their spiritual journeys of self-improvement and self-realization.

It is Acharya Shree's mission to spread the message of nonviolence, vegetarianism, oneness, and total transformation.

CONNECT WITH US

Acharya Shree Yogeesh

http://acharyashreeyogeesh.com

Siddhayatan Spiritual Retreat Center
http://siddhayatan.org

9985 E. Hwy 56
Windom, Texas 75492
info@siddhayatan.org
903.487.0717

Acharya Shree Yogeesh's YouTube Channels
http://youtube.com/yogeeshashram
http://youtube.com/siddhayatan

Acharya Shree Yogeesh's Facebook Fan Page
https://facebook.com/AcharyaShreeYogeesh

Acharya Shree Yogeesh on Instagram
http://instagram.com/AcharyaShreeYogeesh

CPSIA information can be obtained
at www.ICGtesting.com
Printed in the USA
JSHW030354241020
8969JS00003B/8